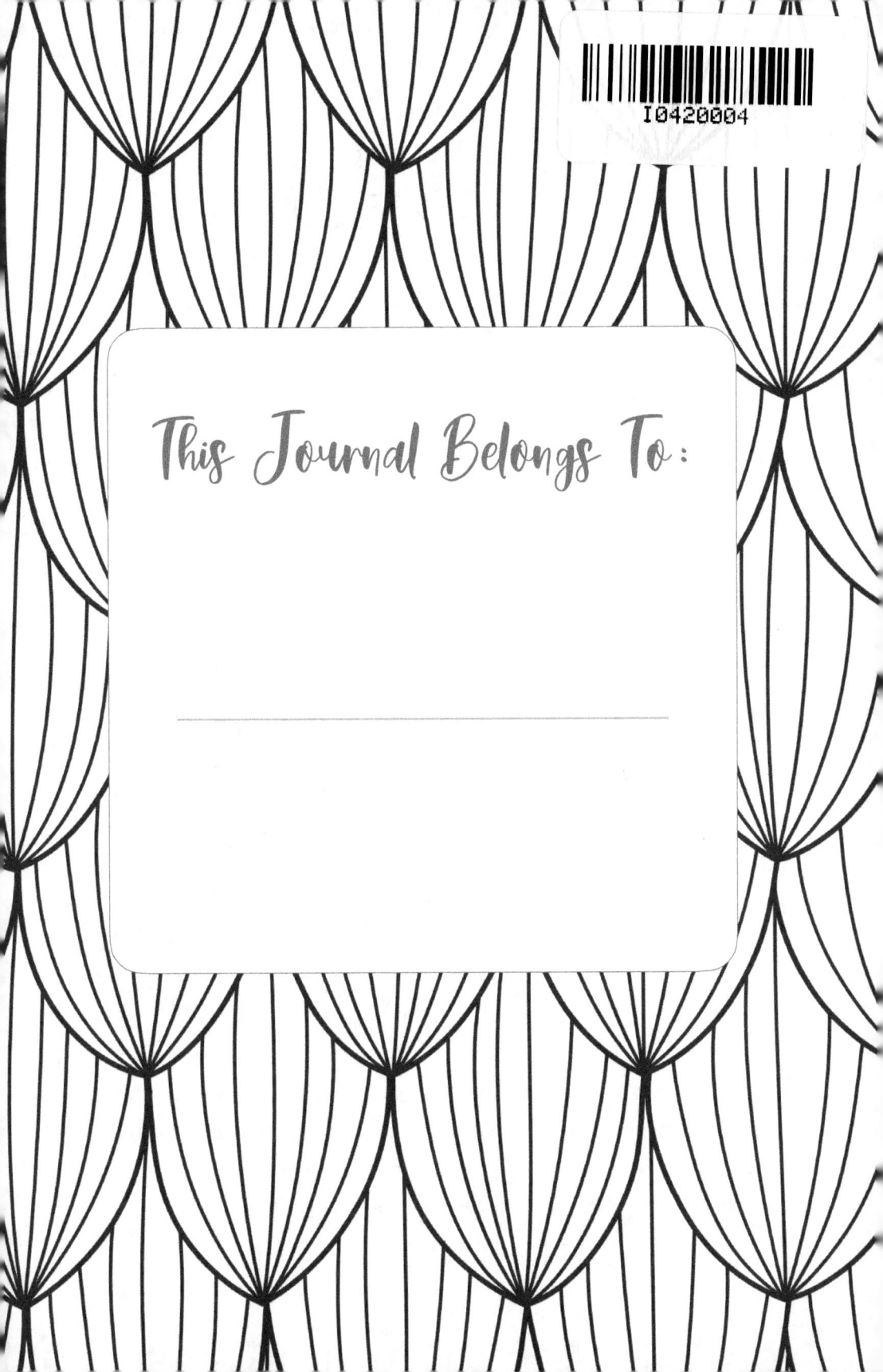

This Journal Belongs To:

_____

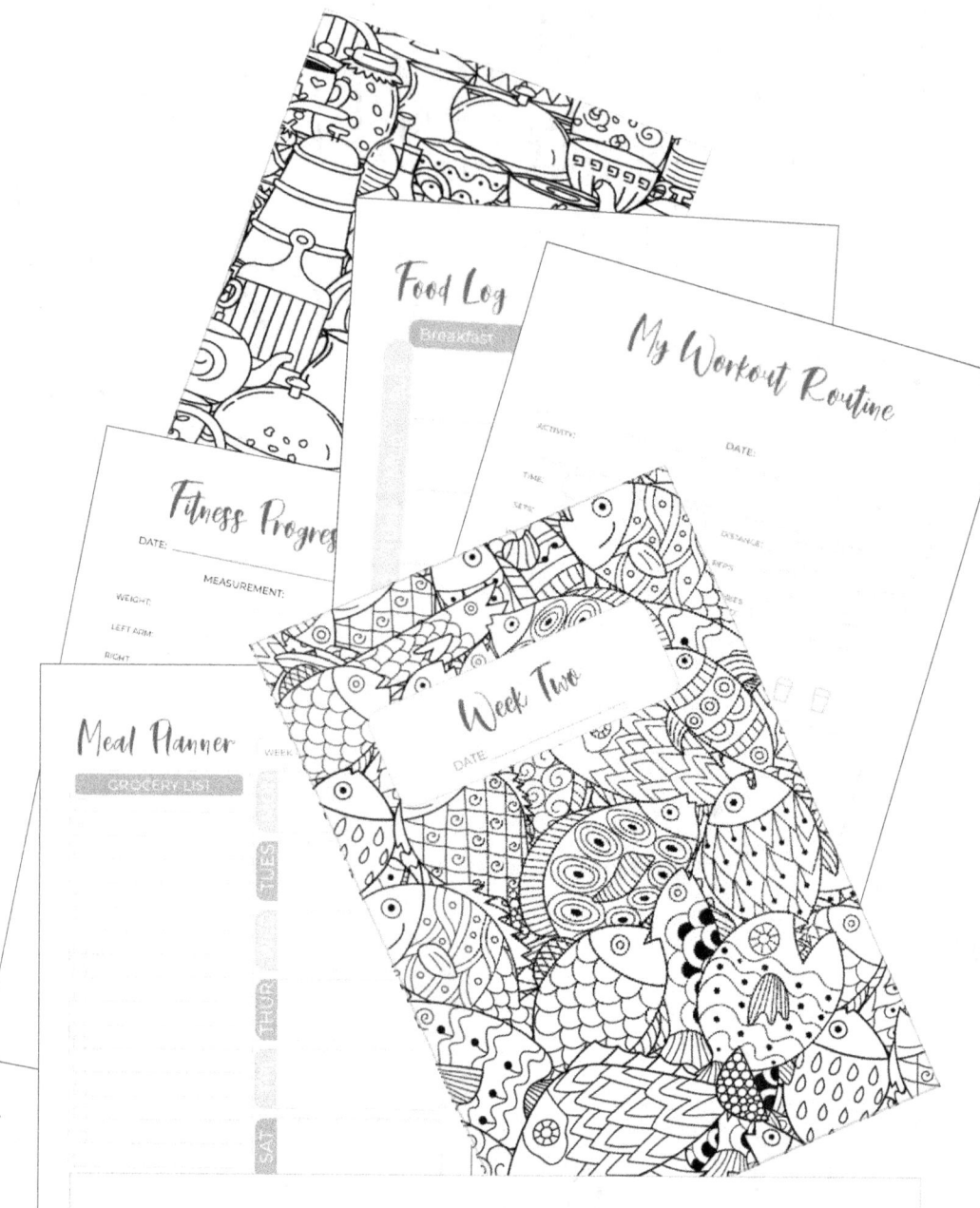

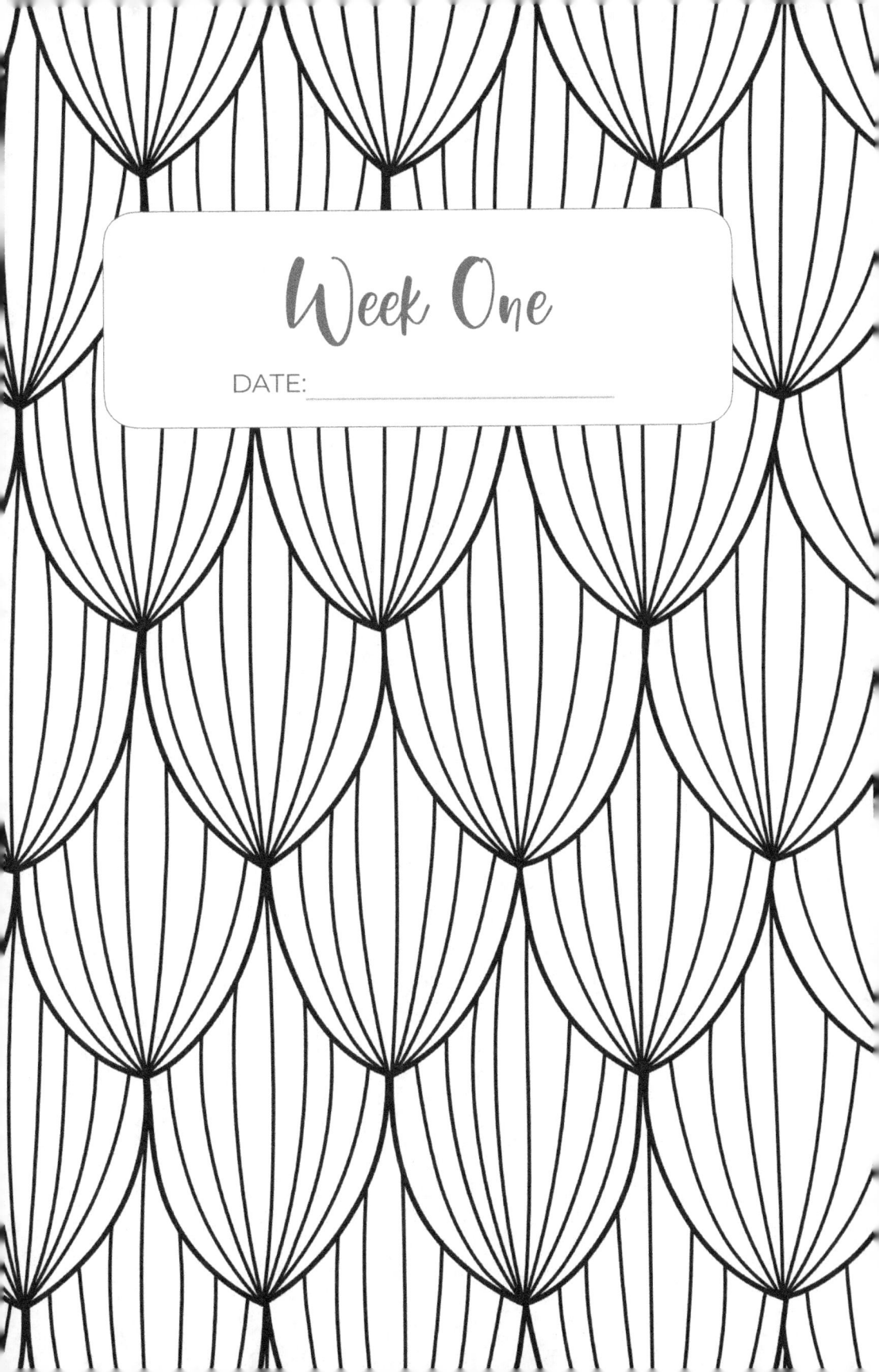

Week One

DATE: _____

This Week's Goals

FITNESS TO DO   **M   T   W   T   F   S   S**

Fitness Progress Tracker

STARTING MEASUREMENTS

DATE: _____

WEIGHT +/-

_____
LEFT BICEP

_____
CHEST

_____
RIGHT BICEP

_____
WAIST

_____
HIPS

_____
LEFT THIGH

_____
RIGHT THIGH

_____
LEFT CALF

_____
RIGHT CALF

My Workout Routine

DATE:

ACTIVITY:

TIME:

DISTANCE:

SETS:

REPS:

WEIGHT USED:

CALORIES BURNED:

WATER INTAKE:

NOTES:

Just Breathe

My Workout Routine

DATE:

ACTIVITY:

TIME:

DISTANCE:

SETS:

REPS:

WEIGHT USED:

CALORIES BURNED:

WATER INTAKE:

NOTES:

Just Breathe

My Workout Routine

DATE:

ACTIVITY:

TIME:

DISTANCE:

SETS:

REPS:

WEIGHT USED:

CALORIES BURNED:

WATER INTAKE:

NOTES:

Just Breathe

My Workout Routine

DATE:

ACTIVITY:

TIME:

DISTANCE:

SETS:

REPS:

WEIGHT USED:

CALORIES BURNED:

WATER INTAKE:

NOTES:

Just Breathe

Meal Planner

WEEK OF

GROCERY LIST

- [ ]
- [ ]
- [ ]
- [ ]
- [ ]
- [ ]
- [ ]
- [ ]
- [ ]
- [ ]
- [ ]
- [ ]
- [ ]
- [ ]
- [ ]
- [ ]
- [ ]
- [ ]
- [ ]
- [ ]
- [ ]

MON

TUES

WED

THUR

FRI

SAT

SUN

Food Log

WEEK OF

	Breakfast	Lunch	Dinner	Snacks
Sun				
Mon				
Tues				
Wed				
Thur				
Fri				
Sat				

Thoughts. . .

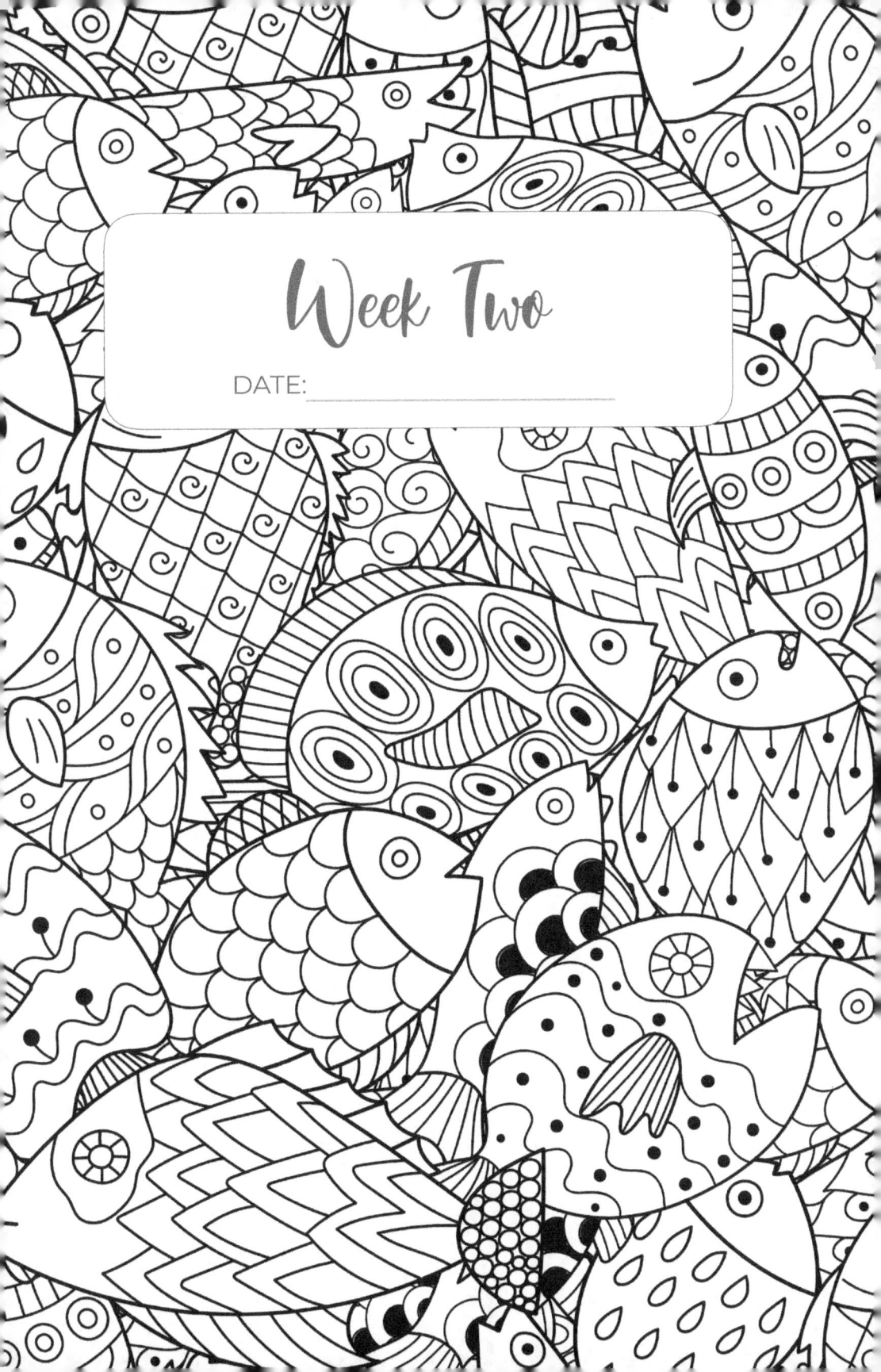

Week Two

DATE: _____

This Week's Goals

FITNESS TO DO	M	T	W	T	F	S	S
	○	○	○	○	○	○	○
	○	○	○	○	○	○	○
	○	○	○	○	○	○	○
	○	○	○	○	○	○	○
	○	○	○	○	○	○	○
	○	○	○	○	○	○	○
	○	○	○	○	○	○	○
	○	○	○	○	○	○	○
	○	○	○	○	○	○	○
	○	○	○	○	○	○	○
	○	○	○	○	○	○	○
	○	○	○	○	○	○	○
	○	○	○	○	○	○	○
	○	○	○	○	○	○	○
	○	○	○	○	○	○	○

Fitness Progress Tracker

DATE: _____

	MEASUREMENT:	LOSS/GAIN:
WEIGHT:		
LEFT ARM:		
RIGHT ARM:		
CHEST:		
WAIST:		
HIPS:		
LEFT THIGH:		
RIGHT THIGH:		

How's It Going?

Good things TAKE TIME

My Workout Routine

DATE:

ACTIVITY:

TIME:

DISTANCE:

SETS:

REPS:

WEIGHT USED:

CALORIES BURNED:

WATER INTAKE:

NOTES:

Just Breathe

My Workout Routine

DATE:

ACTIVITY:

TIME:

DISTANCE:

SETS:

REPS:

WEIGHT USED:

CALORIES BURNED:

WATER INTAKE:

NOTES:

Just Breathe

My Workout Routine

DATE:

ACTIVITY:

TIME:

DISTANCE:

SETS:

REPS:

WEIGHT USED:

CALORIES BURNED:

WATER INTAKE:

NOTES:

Just Breathe

My Workout Routine

DATE:

ACTIVITY:

TIME:

DISTANCE:

SETS:

REPS:

WEIGHT USED:

CALORIES BURNED:

WATER INTAKE:

NOTES:

Just Breathe

Meal Planner

GROCERY LIST

- [ ] _____
- [ ] _____
- [ ] _____
- [ ] _____
- [ ] _____
- [ ] _____
- [ ] _____
- [ ] _____
- [ ] _____
- [ ] _____
- [ ] _____
- [ ] _____
- [ ] _____
- [ ] _____
- [ ] _____
- [ ] _____
- [ ] _____
- [ ] _____
- [ ] _____
- [ ] _____

MON

TUES

WED

THUR

FRI

SAT

SUN

Food Log

WEEK OF

	Breakfast	Lunch	Dinner	Snacks
Sun				
Mon				
Tues				
Wed				
Thur				
Fri				
Sat				

Thoughts. . .

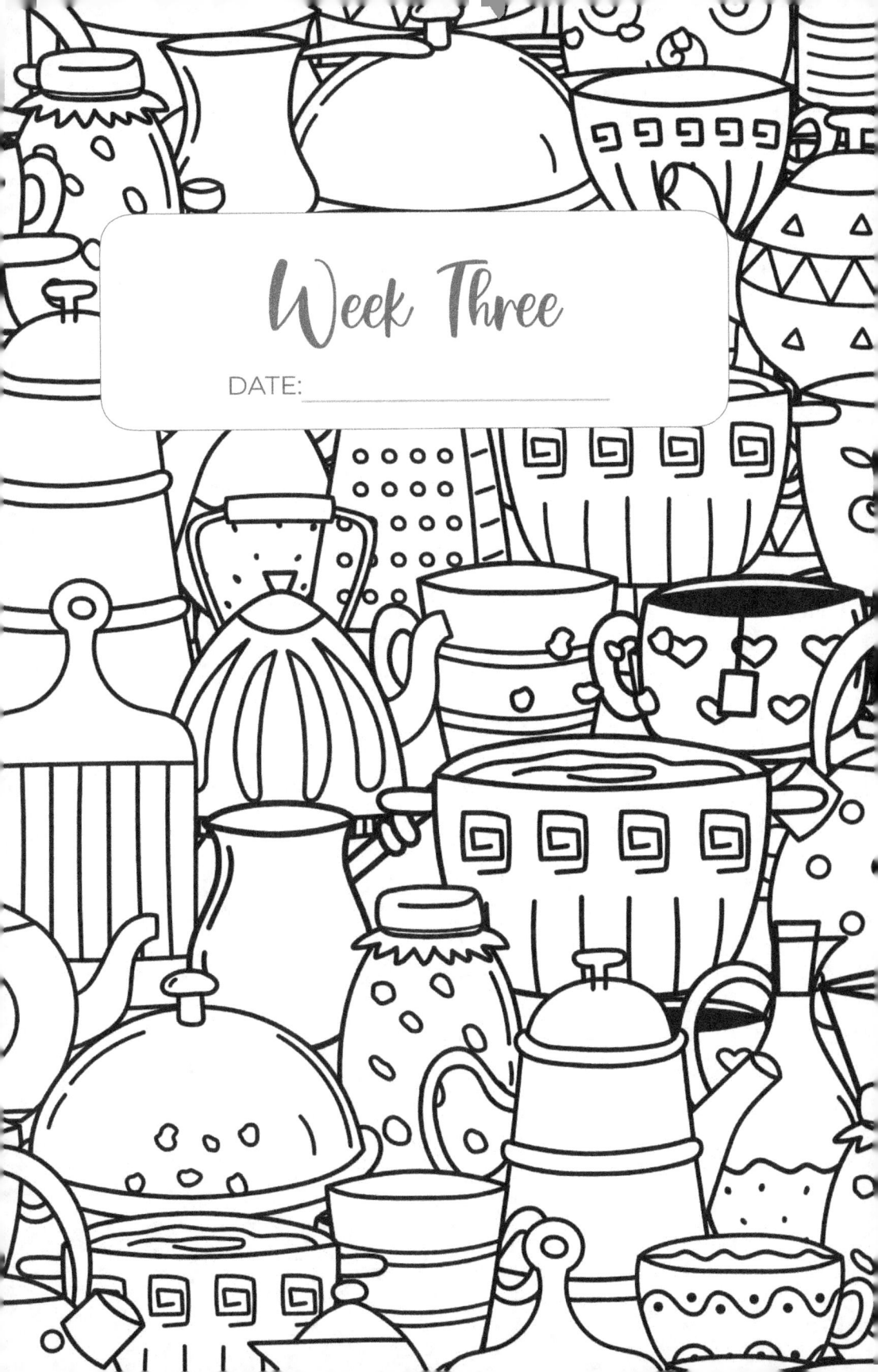

Week Three

DATE: _____

This Week's Goals

FITNESS TO DO   M   T   W   T   F   S   S

Fitness Progress Tracker

DATE: _____

	MEASUREMENT:	LOSS/GAIN:
WEIGHT:		
LEFT ARM:		
RIGHT ARM:		
CHEST:		
WAIST:		
HIPS:		
LEFT THIGH:		
RIGHT THIGH:		

How's It Going?

Good things TAKE TIME

My Workout Routine

DATE:

ACTIVITY:

TIME:

DISTANCE:

SETS:

REPS:

WEIGHT USED:

CALORIES BURNED:

WATER INTAKE:

NOTES:

Just Breathe

My Workout Routine

DATE:

ACTIVITY:

TIME:

DISTANCE:

SETS:

REPS:

WEIGHT USED:

CALORIES BURNED:

WATER INTAKE:

NOTES:

Just Breathe

My Workout Routine

DATE:

ACTIVITY:

TIME:

DISTANCE:

SETS:

REPS:

WEIGHT USED:

CALORIES BURNED:

WATER INTAKE:

NOTES:

Just Breathe

My Workout Routine

DATE:

ACTIVITY:

TIME:

DISTANCE:

SETS:

REPS:

WEIGHT USED:

CALORIES BURNED:

WATER INTAKE:

NOTES:

Just Breathe

Meal Planner

WEEK OF

GROCERY LIST

- [ ]
- [ ]
- [ ]
- [ ]
- [ ]
- [ ]
- [ ]
- [ ]
- [ ]
- [ ]
- [ ]
- [ ]
- [ ]
- [ ]
- [ ]
- [ ]
- [ ]
- [ ]
- [ ]
- [ ]

MON

TUES

WED

THUR

FRI

SAT

SUN

Food Log

WEEK OF

	Breakfast	Lunch	Dinner	Snacks
Sun				
Mon				
Tues				
Wed				
Thur				
Fri				
Sat				

Thoughts. . .

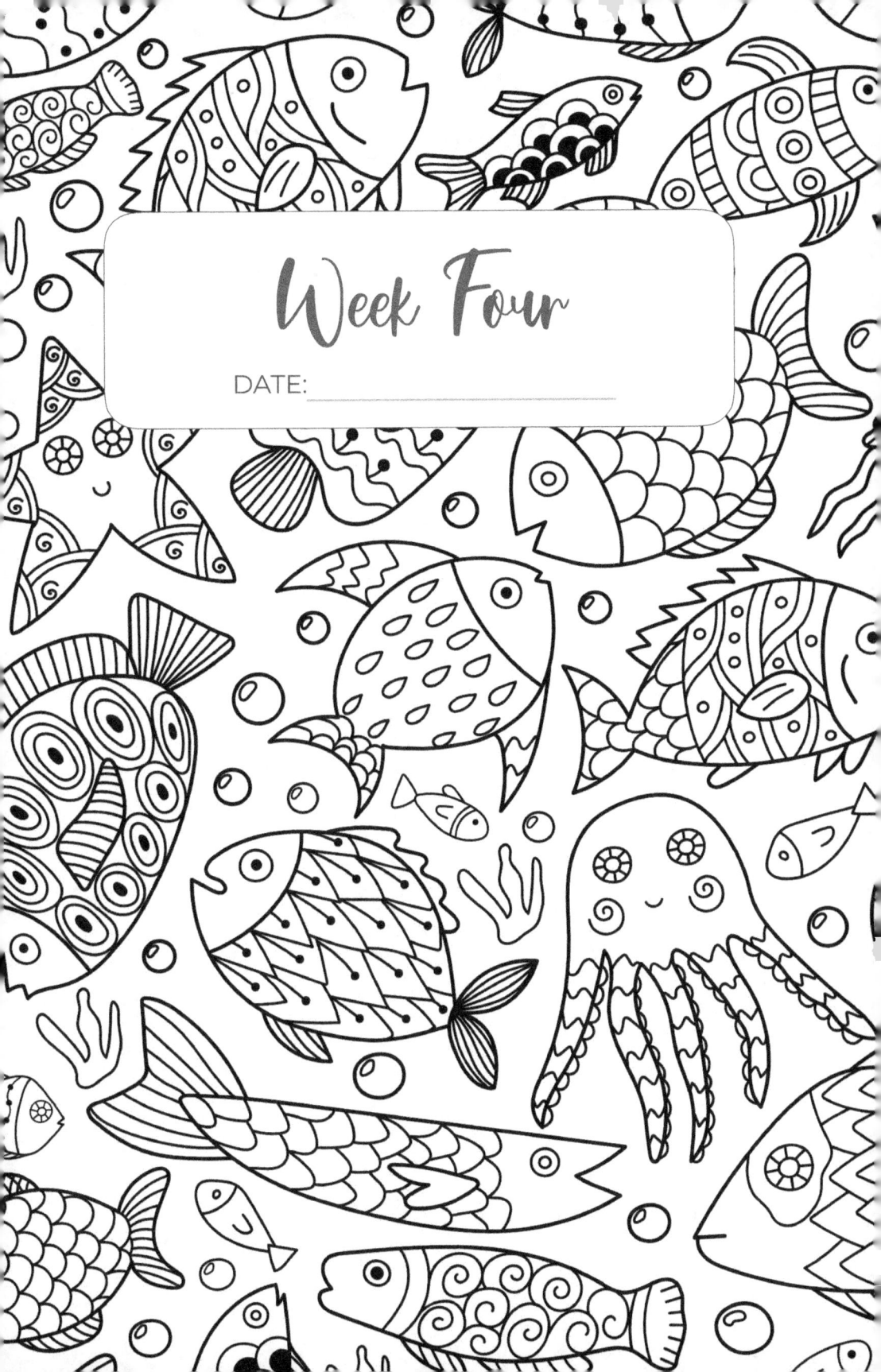

Week Four

DATE: _____

This Week's Goals

FITNESS TO DO   M T W T F S S

Fitness Progress Tracker

DATE: _____

	MEASUREMENT:	LOSS/GAIN:
WEIGHT:		
LEFT ARM:		
RIGHT ARM:		
CHEST:		
WAIST:		
HIPS:		
LEFT THIGH:		
RIGHT THIGH:		

How's It Going?

Good things TAKE TIME

My Workout Routine

DATE:

ACTIVITY:

TIME:

DISTANCE:

SETS:

REPS:

WEIGHT USED:

CALORIES BURNED:

WATER INTAKE:

NOTES:

Just Breathe

My Workout Routine

DATE:

ACTIVITY:

TIME:

DISTANCE:

SETS:

REPS:

WEIGHT USED:

CALORIES BURNED:

WATER INTAKE:

NOTES:

Just Breathe

My Workout Routine

DATE:

ACTIVITY:

TIME:

DISTANCE:

SETS:

REPS:

WEIGHT USED:

CALORIES BURNED:

WATER INTAKE:

NOTES:

Just Breathe

My Workout Routine

DATE:

ACTIVITY:

TIME:

DISTANCE:

SETS:

REPS:

WEIGHT USED:

CALORIES BURNED:

WATER INTAKE:

NOTES:

Just Breathe

Meal Planner

WEEK OF

GROCERY LIST

- [ ]
- [ ]
- [ ]
- [ ]
- [ ]
- [ ]
- [ ]
- [ ]
- [ ]
- [ ]
- [ ]
- [ ]
- [ ]
- [ ]
- [ ]
- [ ]
- [ ]
- [ ]

MON

TUES

WED

THUR

FRI

SAT

SUN

Food Log

WEEK OF

	Breakfast	Lunch	Dinner	Snacks
Sun				
Mon				
Tues				
Wed				
Thur				
Fri				
Sat				

Thoughts. . .

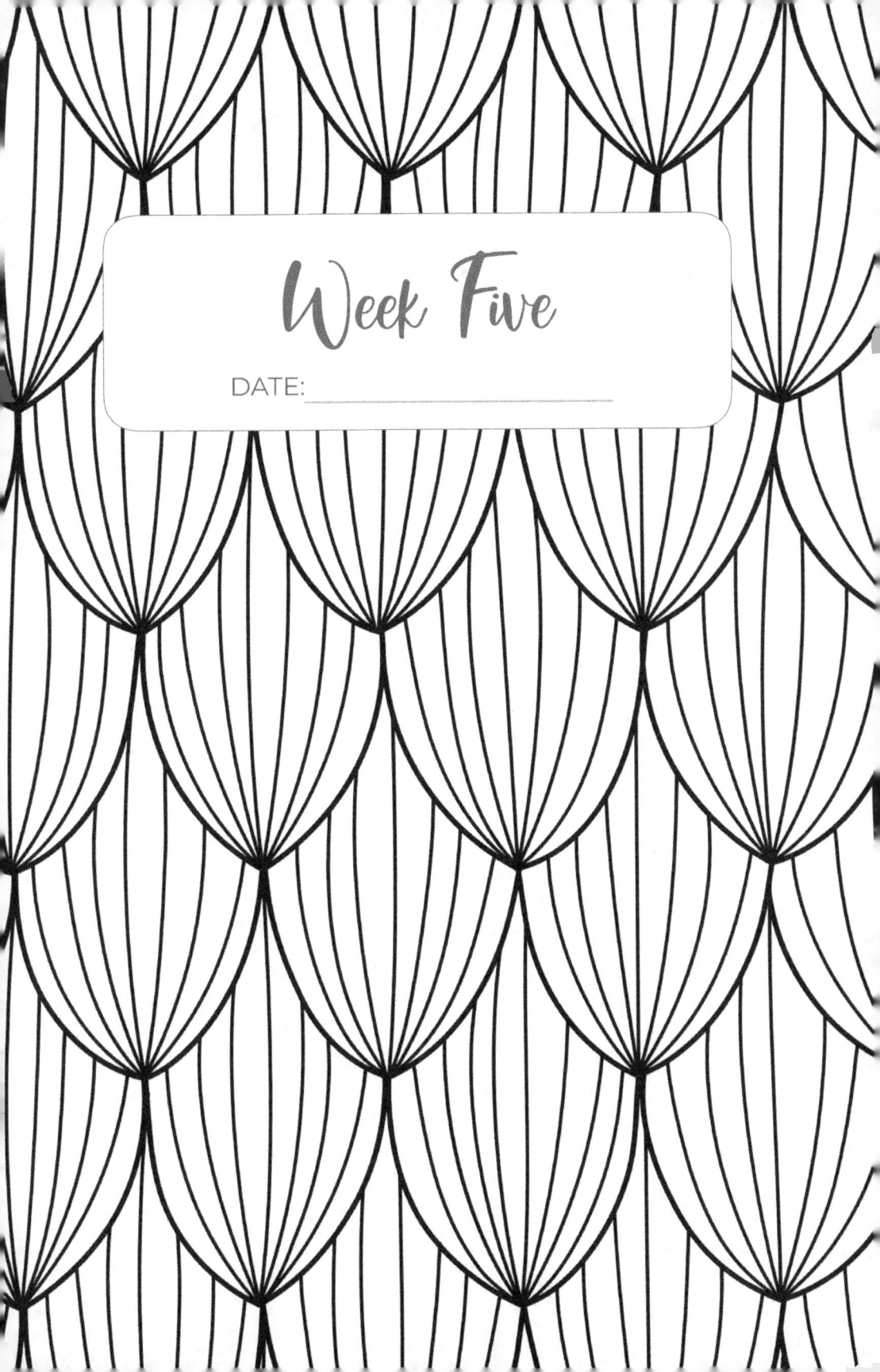

Week Five

DATE: _____

This Week's Goals

FITNESS TO DO   M   T   W   T   F   S   S

Fitness Progress Tracker

DATE: _____

	MEASUREMENT:	LOSS/GAIN:
WEIGHT:		
LEFT ARM:		
RIGHT ARM:		
CHEST:		
WAIST:		
HIPS:		
LEFT THIGH:		
RIGHT THIGH:		

How's It Going?

Good things TAKE TIME

My Workout Routine

DATE:

ACTIVITY:

TIME:

DISTANCE:

SETS:

REPS:

WEIGHT USED:

CALORIES BURNED:

WATER INTAKE:

NOTES:

Just Breathe

My Workout Routine

DATE:

ACTIVITY:

TIME:

DISTANCE:

SETS:

REPS:

WEIGHT USED:

CALORIES BURNED:

WATER INTAKE:

NOTES:

Just Breathe

My Workout Routine

DATE:

ACTIVITY:

TIME:

DISTANCE:

SETS:

REPS:

WEIGHT USED:

CALORIES BURNED:

WATER INTAKE:

NOTES:

Just Breathe

My Workout Routine

DATE:

ACTIVITY:

TIME:

DISTANCE:

SETS:

REPS:

WEIGHT USED:

CALORIES BURNED:

WATER INTAKE:

NOTES:

Just Breathe

Meal Planner

GROCERY LIST

- [ ]
- [ ]
- [ ]
- [ ]
- [ ]
- [ ]
- [ ]
- [ ]
- [ ]
- [ ]
- [ ]
- [ ]
- [ ]
- [ ]
- [ ]
- [ ]
- [ ]
- [ ]
- [ ]
- [ ]

MON

TUES

WED

THUR

FRI

SAT

SUN

Food Log

WEEK OF

	Breakfast	Lunch	Dinner	Snacks
Sun				
Mon				
Tues				
Wed				
Thur				
Fri				
Sat				

Thoughts. . .

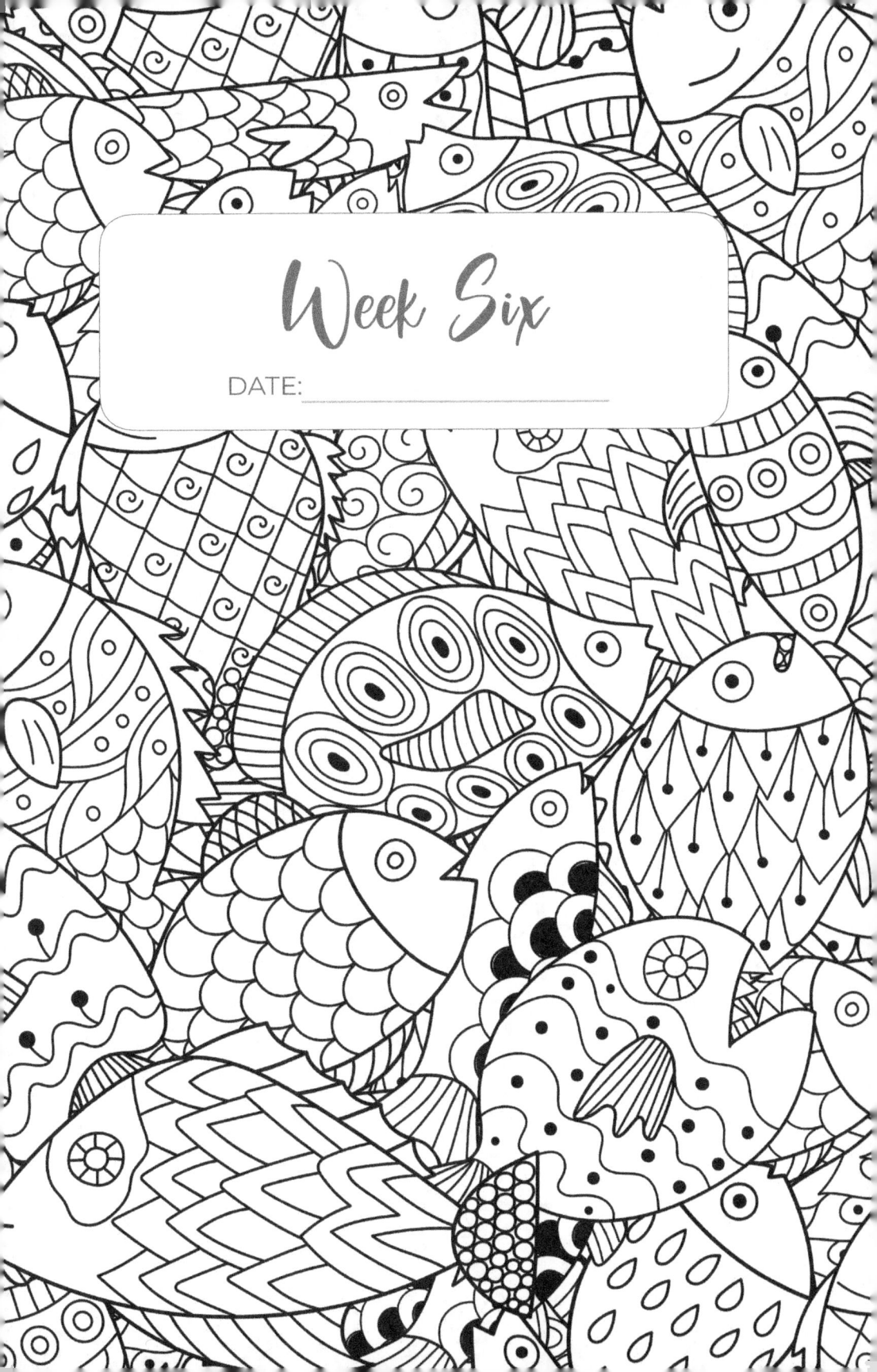

Week Six

DATE: _____

This Week's Goals

FITNESS TO DO   **M**   **T**   **W**   **T**   **F**   **S**   **S**

Fitness Progress Tracker

DATE: _____

	MEASUREMENT:	LOSS/GAIN:
WEIGHT:		
LEFT ARM:		
RIGHT ARM:		
CHEST:		
WAIST:		
HIPS:		
LEFT THIGH:		
RIGHT THIGH:		

How's It Going?

Good things TAKE TIME

My Workout Routine

DATE:

ACTIVITY:

TIME:

DISTANCE:

SETS:

REPS:

WEIGHT USED:

CALORIES BURNED:

WATER INTAKE:

NOTES:

Just Breathe

My Workout Routine

DATE:

ACTIVITY:

TIME:

DISTANCE:

SETS:

REPS:

WEIGHT USED:

CALORIES BURNED:

WATER INTAKE:

NOTES:

Just Breathe

My Workout Routine

DATE:

ACTIVITY:

TIME:

DISTANCE:

SETS:

REPS:

WEIGHT USED:

CALORIES BURNED:

WATER INTAKE:

NOTES:

Just Breathe

My Workout Routine

DATE:

ACTIVITY:

TIME:

DISTANCE:

SETS:

REPS:

WEIGHT USED:

CALORIES BURNED:

WATER INTAKE:

NOTES:

Just Breathe

Meal Planner

WEEK OF

GROCERY LIST

- [ ]
- [ ]
- [ ]
- [ ]
- [ ]
- [ ]
- [ ]
- [ ]
- [ ]
- [ ]
- [ ]
- [ ]
- [ ]
- [ ]
- [ ]
- [ ]
- [ ]
- [ ]
- [ ]
- [ ]
- [ ]

MON

TUES

WED

THUR

FRI

SAT

SUN

Food Log

WEEK OF

	Breakfast	Lunch	Dinner	Snacks
Sun				
Mon				
Tues				
Wed				
Thur				
Fri				
Sat				

Thoughts. . .

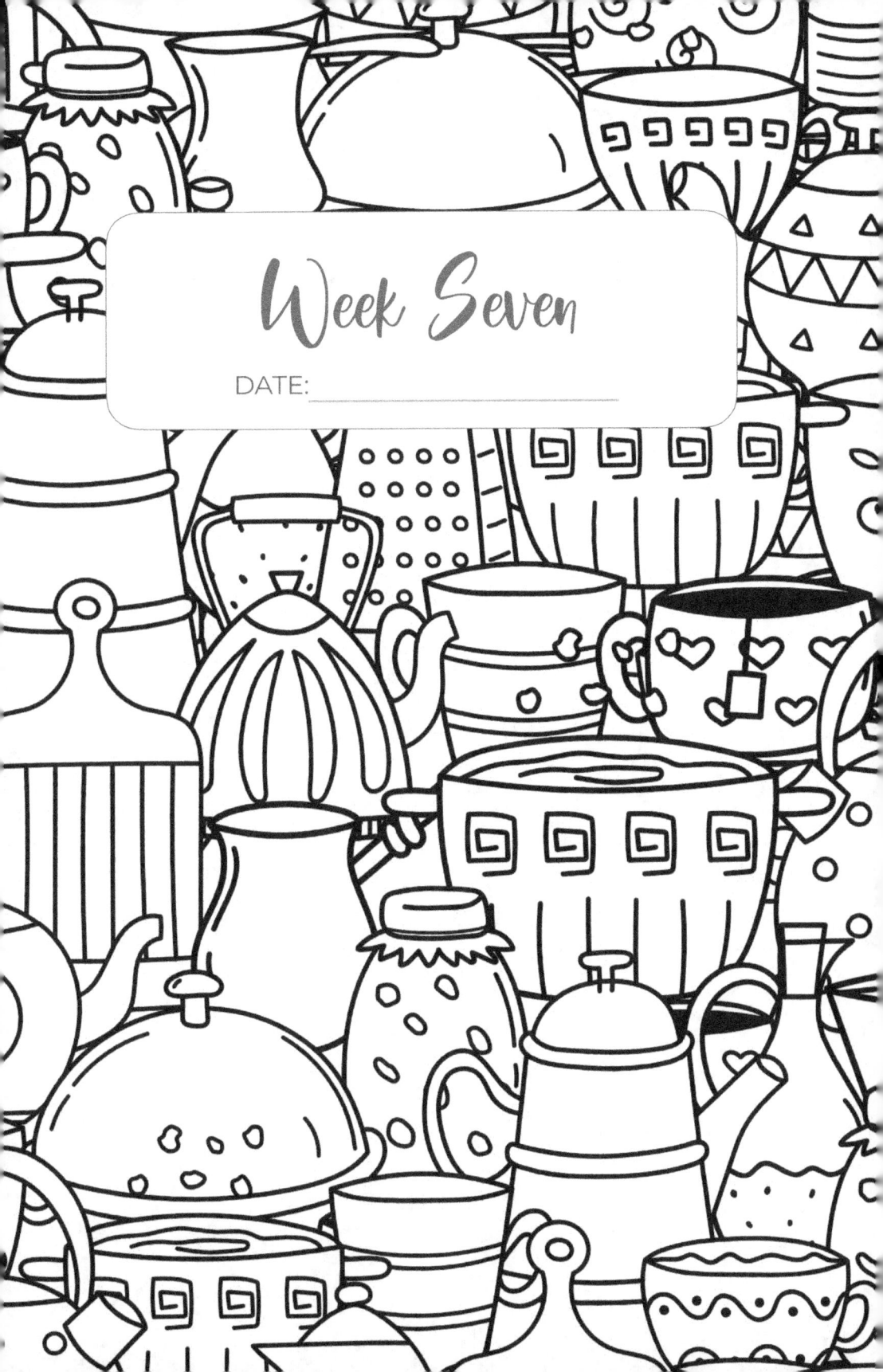

Week Seven

DATE:_____

This Week's Goals

FITNESS TO DO   **M   T   W   T   F   S   S**

Fitness Progress Tracker

DATE: _____

	MEASUREMENT:	LOSS/GAIN:
WEIGHT:		
LEFT ARM:		
RIGHT ARM:		
CHEST:		
WAIST:		
HIPS:		
LEFT THIGH:		
RIGHT THIGH:		

How's It Going?

Good things TAKE TIME

My Workout Routine

DATE:

ACTIVITY:

TIME:

DISTANCE:

SETS:

REPS:

WEIGHT USED:

CALORIES BURNED:

WATER INTAKE:

NOTES:

Just Breathe

My Workout Routine

DATE:

ACTIVITY:

TIME:

DISTANCE:

SETS:

REPS:

WEIGHT USED:

CALORIES BURNED:

WATER INTAKE:

NOTES:

Just Breathe

My Workout Routine

DATE:

ACTIVITY:

TIME:

DISTANCE:

SETS:

REPS:

WEIGHT USED:

CALORIES BURNED:

WATER INTAKE:

NOTES:

Just Breathe

My Workout Routine

DATE:

ACTIVITY:

TIME:

DISTANCE:

SETS:

REPS:

WEIGHT
USED:

CALORIES
BURNED:

WATER INTAKE:

NOTES:

Just
Breathe

Meal Planner

WEEK OF

GROCERY LIST

- [ ]
- [ ]
- [ ]
- [ ]
- [ ]
- [ ]
- [ ]
- [ ]
- [ ]
- [ ]
- [ ]
- [ ]
- [ ]
- [ ]
- [ ]
- [ ]
- [ ]
- [ ]
- [ ]

MON

TUES

WED

THUR

FRI

SAT

SUN

Food Log

	Breakfast	Lunch	Dinner	Snacks
Sun				
Mon				
Tues				
Wed				
Thur				
Fri				
Sat				

Thoughts. . .

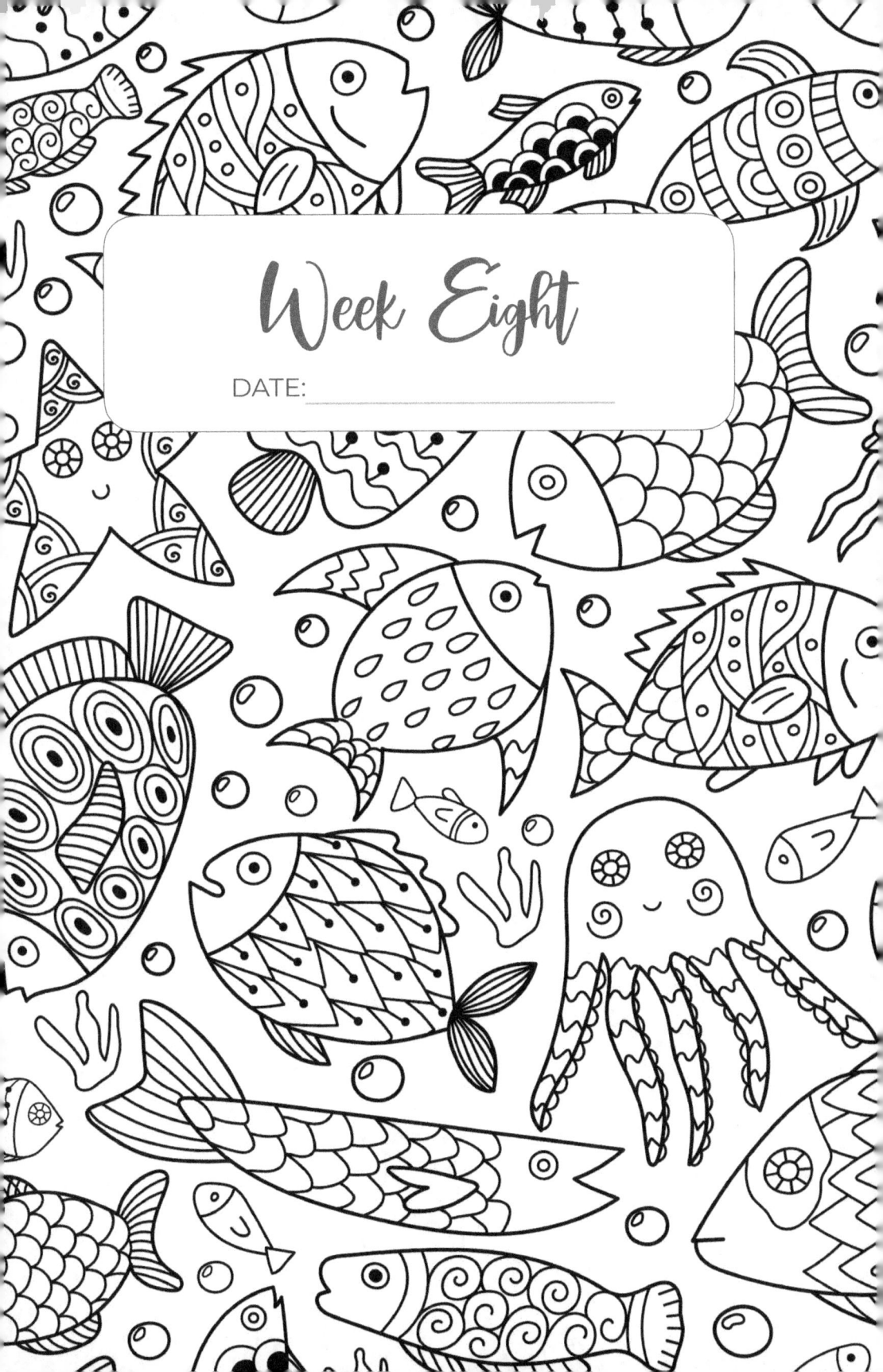

Week Eight

DATE:_____

This Week's Goals

FITNESS TO DO   M   T   W   T   F   S   S

Fitness Progress Tracker

DATE: _____

	MEASUREMENT:	LOSS/GAIN:
WEIGHT:		
LEFT ARM:		
RIGHT ARM:		
CHEST:		
WAIST:		
HIPS:		
LEFT THIGH:		
RIGHT THIGH:		

How's It Going?

Good things TAKE TIME

My Workout Routine

DATE:

ACTIVITY:

TIME:

DISTANCE:

SETS:

REPS:

WEIGHT USED:

CALORIES BURNED:

WATER INTAKE:

NOTES:

Just Breathe

My Workout Routine

DATE:

ACTIVITY:

TIME:

DISTANCE:

SETS:

REPS:

WEIGHT USED:

CALORIES BURNED:

WATER INTAKE:

NOTES:

Just Breathe

My Workout Routine

DATE:

ACTIVITY:

TIME:

DISTANCE:

SETS:

REPS:

WEIGHT USED:

CALORIES BURNED:

WATER INTAKE:

NOTES:

Just Breathe

My Workout Routine

DATE:

ACTIVITY:

TIME:

DISTANCE:

SETS:

REPS:

WEIGHT USED:

CALORIES BURNED:

WATER INTAKE:

NOTES:

Just Breathe

Meal Planner

WEEK OF

GROCERY LIST

- [ ]
- [ ]
- [ ]
- [ ]
- [ ]
- [ ]
- [ ]
- [ ]
- [ ]
- [ ]
- [ ]
- [ ]
- [ ]
- [ ]
- [ ]
- [ ]
- [ ]
- [ ]
- [ ]
- [ ]

MON

TUES

WED

THUR

FRI

SAT

SUN

Food Log

WEEK OF

	Breakfast	Lunch	Dinner	Snacks
Sun				
Mon				
Tues				
Wed				
Thur				
Fri				
Sat				

Thoughts. . .

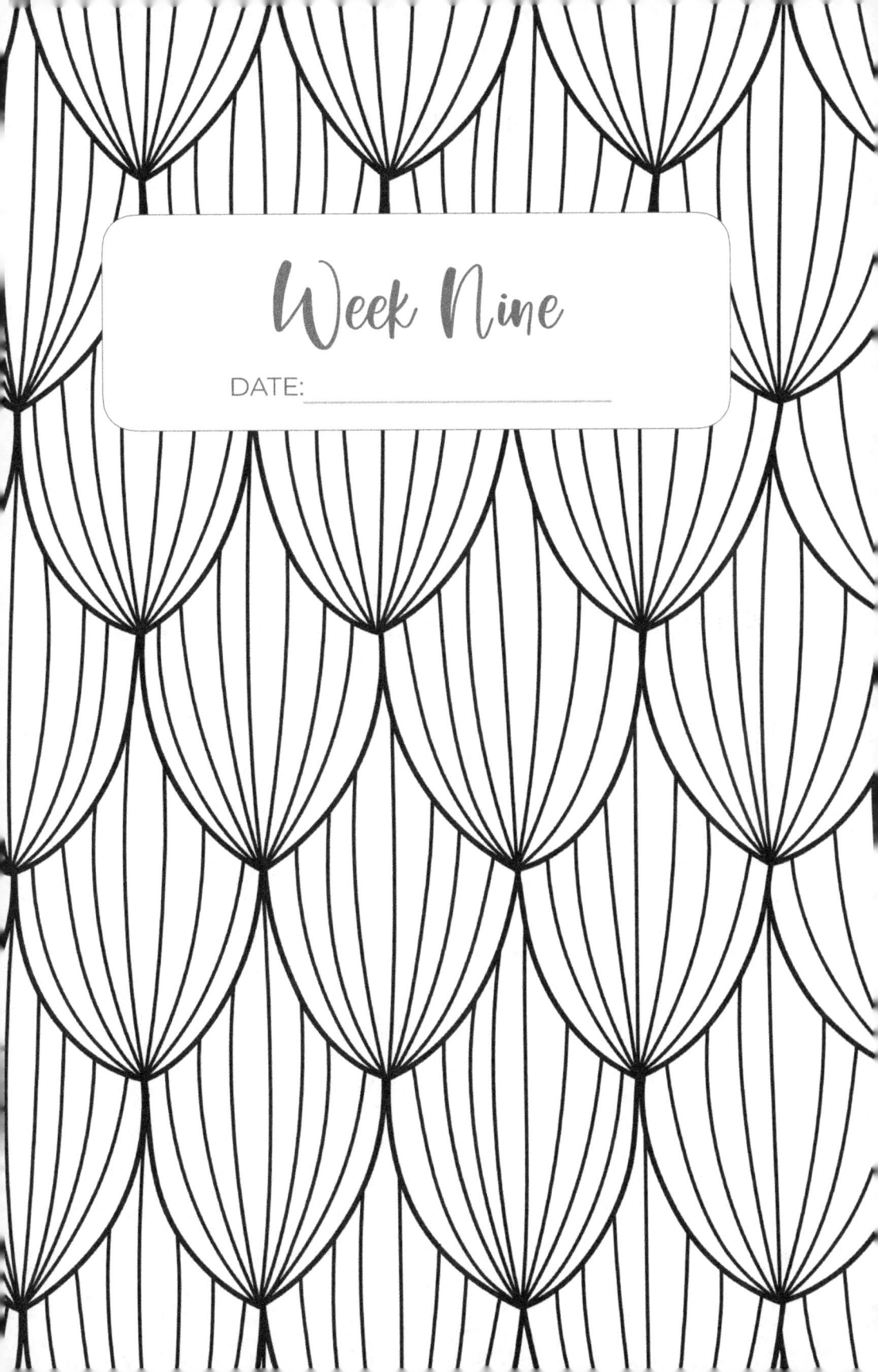

Week Nine

DATE: _____

This Week's Goals

FITNESS TO DO   M   T   W   T   F   S   S

Fitness Progress Tracker

DATE: _____

	MEASUREMENT:	LOSS/GAIN:
WEIGHT:		
LEFT ARM:		
RIGHT ARM:		
CHEST:		
WAIST:		
HIPS:		
LEFT THIGH:		
RIGHT THIGH:		

How's It Going?

Good things TAKE TIME

My Workout Routine

DATE:

ACTIVITY:

TIME:

DISTANCE:

SETS:

REPS:

WEIGHT USED:

CALORIES BURNED:

WATER INTAKE:

NOTES:

Just Breathe

My Workout Routine

DATE:

ACTIVITY:

TIME:

DISTANCE:

SETS:

REPS:

WEIGHT USED:

CALORIES BURNED:

WATER INTAKE:

NOTES:

Just Breathe

My Workout Routine

DATE:

ACTIVITY:

TIME:

DISTANCE:

SETS:

REPS:

WEIGHT USED:

CALORIES BURNED:

WATER INTAKE:

NOTES:

Just Breathe

My Workout Routine

DATE:

ACTIVITY:

TIME:

DISTANCE:

SETS:

REPS:

WEIGHT USED:

CALORIES BURNED:

WATER INTAKE:

NOTES:

Just Breathe

Meal Planner

GROCERY LIST

- ☐
- ☐
- ☐
- ☐
- ☐
- ☐
- ☐
- ☐
- ☐
- ☐
- ☐
- ☐
- ☐
- ☐
- ☐
- ☐
- ☐
- ☐
- ☐
- ☐

MON

TUES

WED

THUR

FRI

SAT

SUN

Food Log

	Breakfast	Lunch	Dinner	Snacks
Sun				
Mon				
Tues				
Wed				
Thur				
Fri				
Sat				

Thoughts. . .

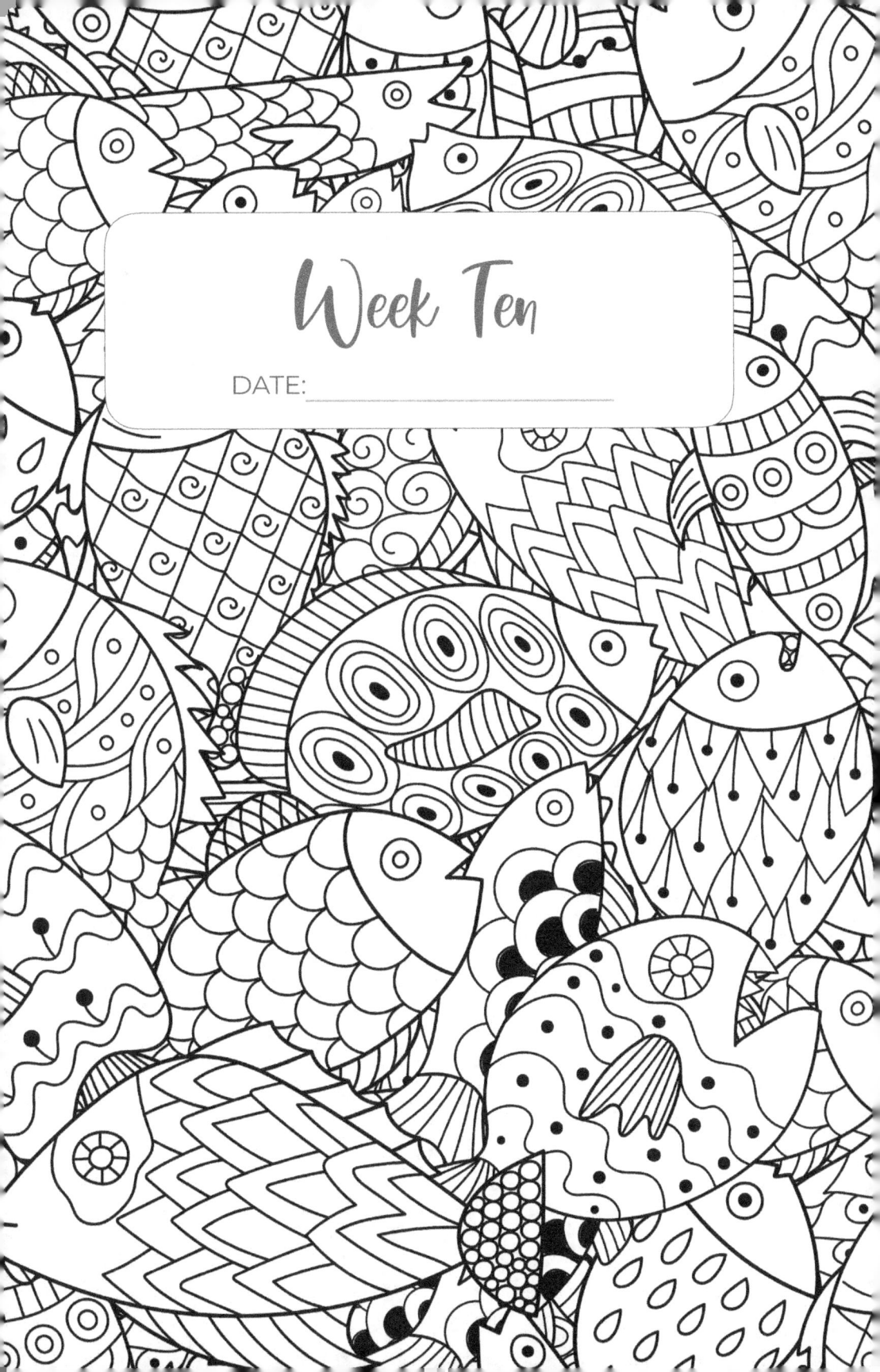

Week Ten

DATE: _____

This Week's Goals

FITNESS TO DO 　　　M　T　W　T　F　S　S

Fitness Progress Tracker

DATE: _____

	MEASUREMENT:	LOSS/GAIN:
WEIGHT:		
LEFT ARM:		
RIGHT ARM:		
CHEST:		
WAIST:		
HIPS:		
LEFT THIGH:		
RIGHT THIGH:		

How's It Going?

Good things TAKE TIME

My Workout Routine

DATE:

ACTIVITY:

TIME:

DISTANCE:

SETS:

REPS:

WEIGHT USED:

CALORIES BURNED:

WATER INTAKE:

NOTES:

Just Breathe

My Workout Routine

DATE:

ACTIVITY:

TIME:

DISTANCE:

SETS:

REPS:

WEIGHT USED:

CALORIES BURNED:

WATER INTAKE:

NOTES:

Just Breathe

My Workout Routine

DATE:

ACTIVITY:

TIME:

DISTANCE:

SETS:

REPS:

WEIGHT USED:

CALORIES BURNED:

WATER INTAKE:

NOTES:

Just Breathe

My Workout Routine

DATE:

ACTIVITY:

TIME:

DISTANCE:

SETS:

REPS:

WEIGHT USED:

CALORIES BURNED:

WATER INTAKE:

NOTES:

Just Breathe

Meal Planner

WEEK OF

GROCERY LIST

MON

TUES

WED

THUR

FRI

SAT

SUN

Food Log

WEEK OF

	Breakfast	Lunch	Dinner	Snacks
Sun				
Mon				
Tues				
Wed				
Thur				
Fri				
Sat				

Thoughts. . .

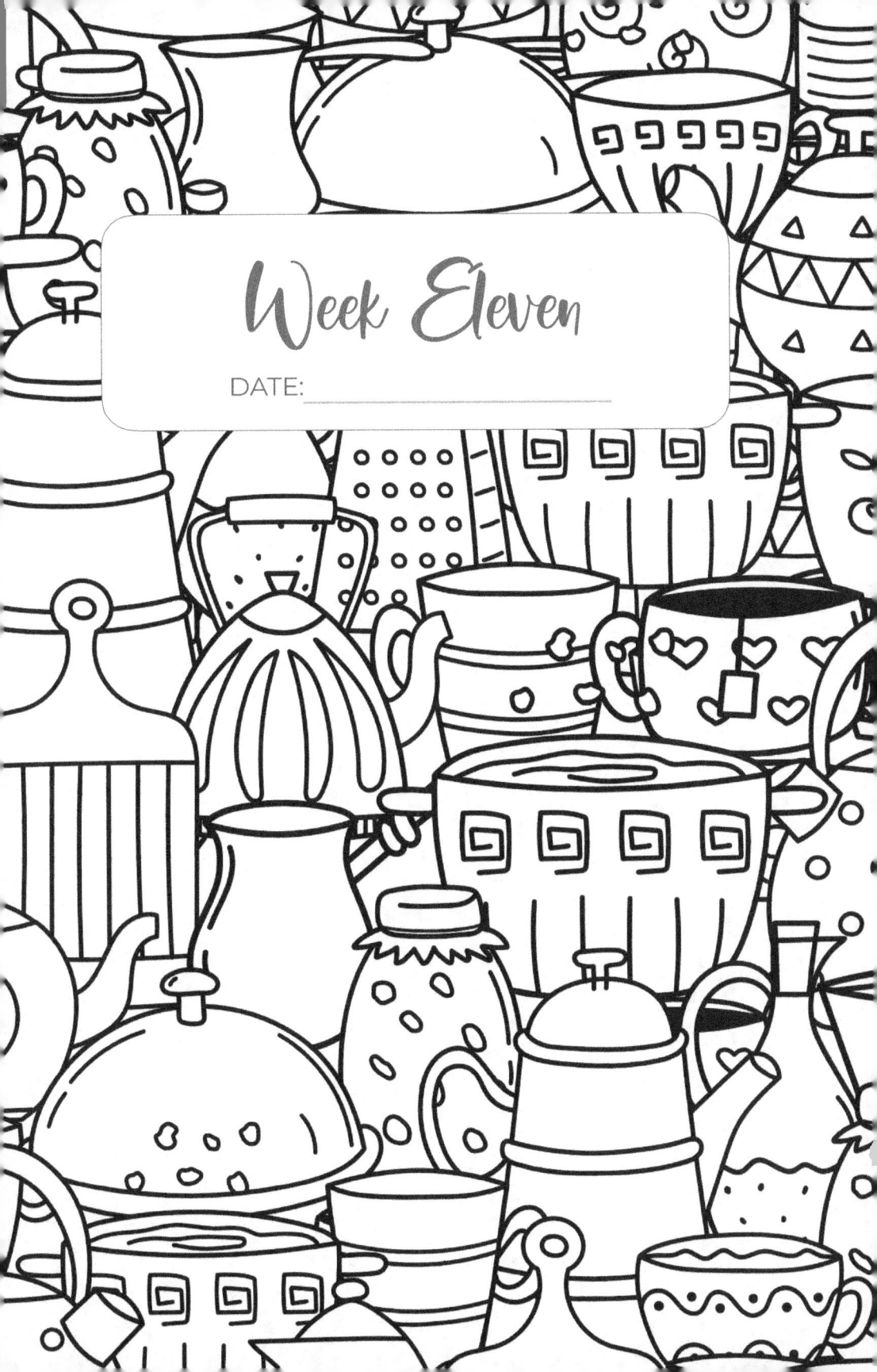

Week Eleven

DATE: _____

This Week's Goals

FITNESS TO DO   **M**   **T**   **W**   **T**   **F**   **S**   **S**

Fitness Progress Tracker

DATE: _____

	MEASUREMENT:	LOSS/GAIN:
WEIGHT:		
LEFT ARM:		
RIGHT ARM:		
CHEST:		
WAIST:		
HIPS:		
LEFT THIGH:		
RIGHT THIGH:		

How's It Going?

Good things TAKE TIME

My Workout Routine

DATE:

ACTIVITY:

TIME:

DISTANCE:

SETS:

REPS:

WEIGHT USED:

CALORIES BURNED:

WATER INTAKE:

NOTES:

Just Breathe

My Workout Routine

DATE:

ACTIVITY:

TIME:

DISTANCE:

SETS:

REPS:

WEIGHT USED:

CALORIES BURNED:

WATER INTAKE:

NOTES:

Just Breathe

My Workout Routine

DATE:

ACTIVITY:

TIME:

DISTANCE:

SETS:

REPS:

WEIGHT USED:

CALORIES BURNED:

WATER INTAKE:

NOTES:

Just Breathe

My Workout Routine

DATE:

ACTIVITY:

TIME:

DISTANCE:

SETS:

REPS:

WEIGHT USED:

CALORIES BURNED:

WATER INTAKE:

NOTES:

Just Breathe

Meal Planner

WEEK OF

GROCERY LIST

- [ ]
- [ ]
- [ ]
- [ ]
- [ ]
- [ ]
- [ ]
- [ ]
- [ ]
- [ ]
- [ ]
- [ ]
- [ ]
- [ ]
- [ ]
- [ ]
- [ ]
- [ ]
- [ ]

MON

TUES

WED

THUR

FRI

SAT

SUN

Food Log

WEEK OF

	Breakfast	Lunch	Dinner	Snacks
Sun				
Mon				
Tues				
Wed				
Thur				
Fri				
Sat				

Thoughts. . .

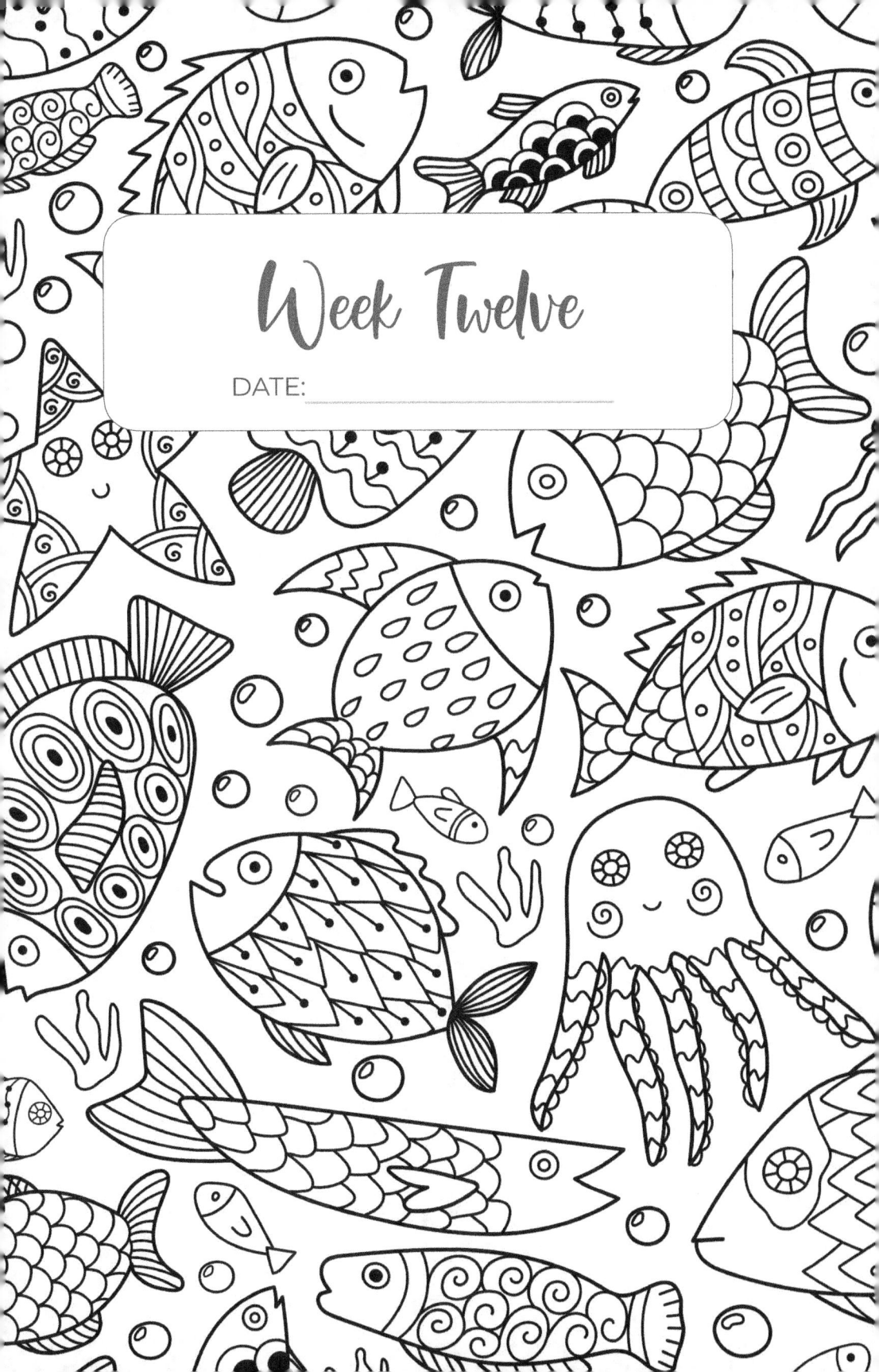

Week Twelve

DATE:

This Week's Goals

FITNESS TO DO

	M	T	W	T	F	S	S
	○	○	○	○	○	○	○
	○	○	○	○	○	○	○
	○	○	○	○	○	○	○
	○	○	○	○	○	○	○
	○	○	○	○	○	○	○
	○	○	○	○	○	○	○
	○	○	○	○	○	○	○
	○	○	○	○	○	○	○
	○	○	○	○	○	○	○
	○	○	○	○	○	○	○
	○	○	○	○	○	○	○
	○	○	○	○	○	○	○
	○	○	○	○	○	○	○
	○	○	○	○	○	○	○
	○	○	○	○	○	○	○
	○	○	○	○	○	○	○
	○	○	○	○	○	○	○

Fitness Progress Tracker

DATE: _____

	MEASUREMENT:	LOSS/GAIN:
WEIGHT:		
LEFT ARM:		
RIGHT ARM:		
CHEST:		
WAIST:		
HIPS:		
LEFT THIGH:		
RIGHT THIGH:		

How's It Going?

Good things TAKE TIME

My Workout Routine

DATE:

ACTIVITY:

TIME:

DISTANCE:

SETS:

REPS:

WEIGHT USED:

CALORIES BURNED:

WATER INTAKE:

NOTES:

Just Breathe

My Workout Routine

DATE:

ACTIVITY:

TIME:

DISTANCE:

SETS:

REPS:

WEIGHT USED:

CALORIES BURNED:

WATER INTAKE:

NOTES:

Just Breathe

My Workout Routine

DATE:

ACTIVITY:

TIME:

DISTANCE:

SETS:

REPS:

WEIGHT USED:

CALORIES BURNED:

WATER INTAKE:

NOTES:

Just Breathe

My Workout Routine

DATE:

ACTIVITY:

TIME:

DISTANCE:

SETS:

REPS:

WEIGHT USED:

CALORIES BURNED:

WATER INTAKE:

NOTES:

Just Breathe

Meal Planner

WEEK OF

GROCERY LIST

- [ ]
- [ ]
- [ ]
- [ ]
- [ ]
- [ ]
- [ ]
- [ ]
- [ ]
- [ ]
- [ ]
- [ ]
- [ ]
- [ ]
- [ ]
- [ ]
- [ ]
- [ ]
- [ ]
- [ ]

MON

TUES

WED

THUR

FRI

SAT

SUN

Food Log

	Breakfast	Lunch	Dinner	Snacks
Sun				
Mon				
Tues				
Wed				
Thur				
Fri				
Sat				

Thoughts. . .

12 - Week Total Weight Log

CURRENT:

PREVIOUS:

CHANGE:

NOTES

Good things TAKE TIME

Congratulations!

You Did It!

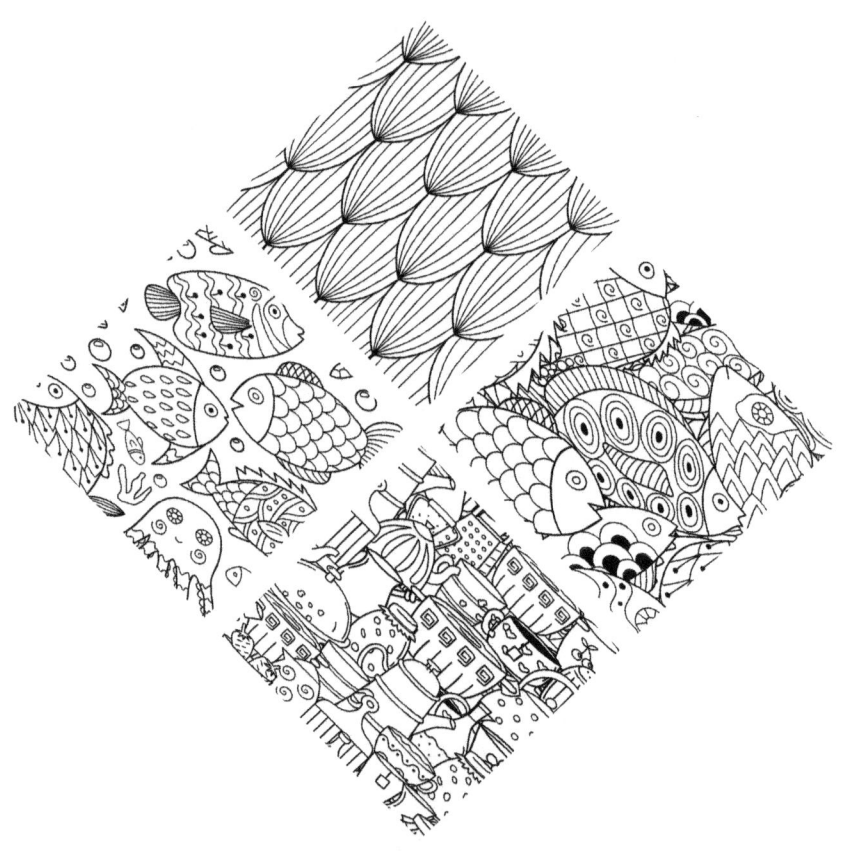

Now It's Time To Play. . .

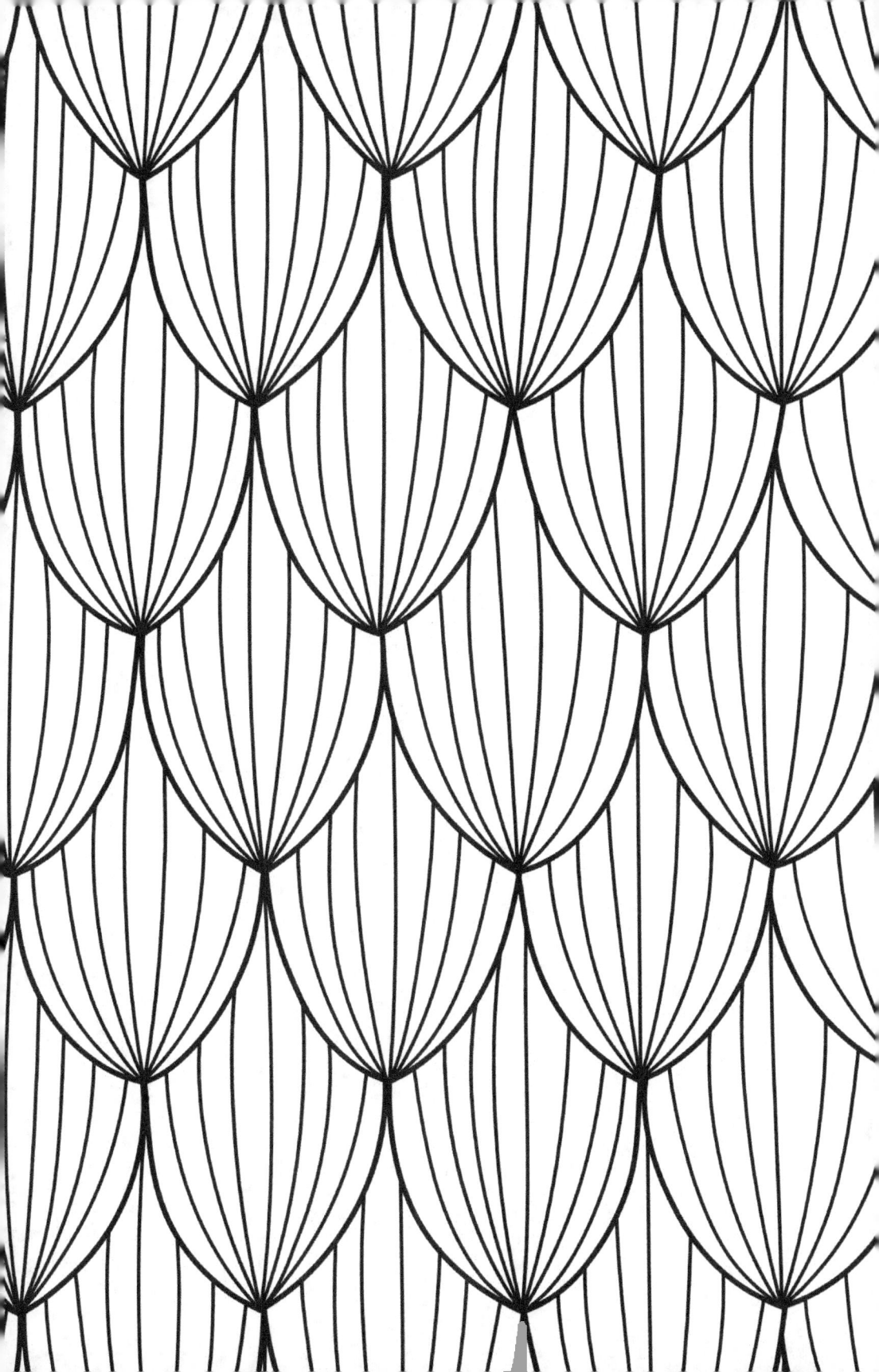

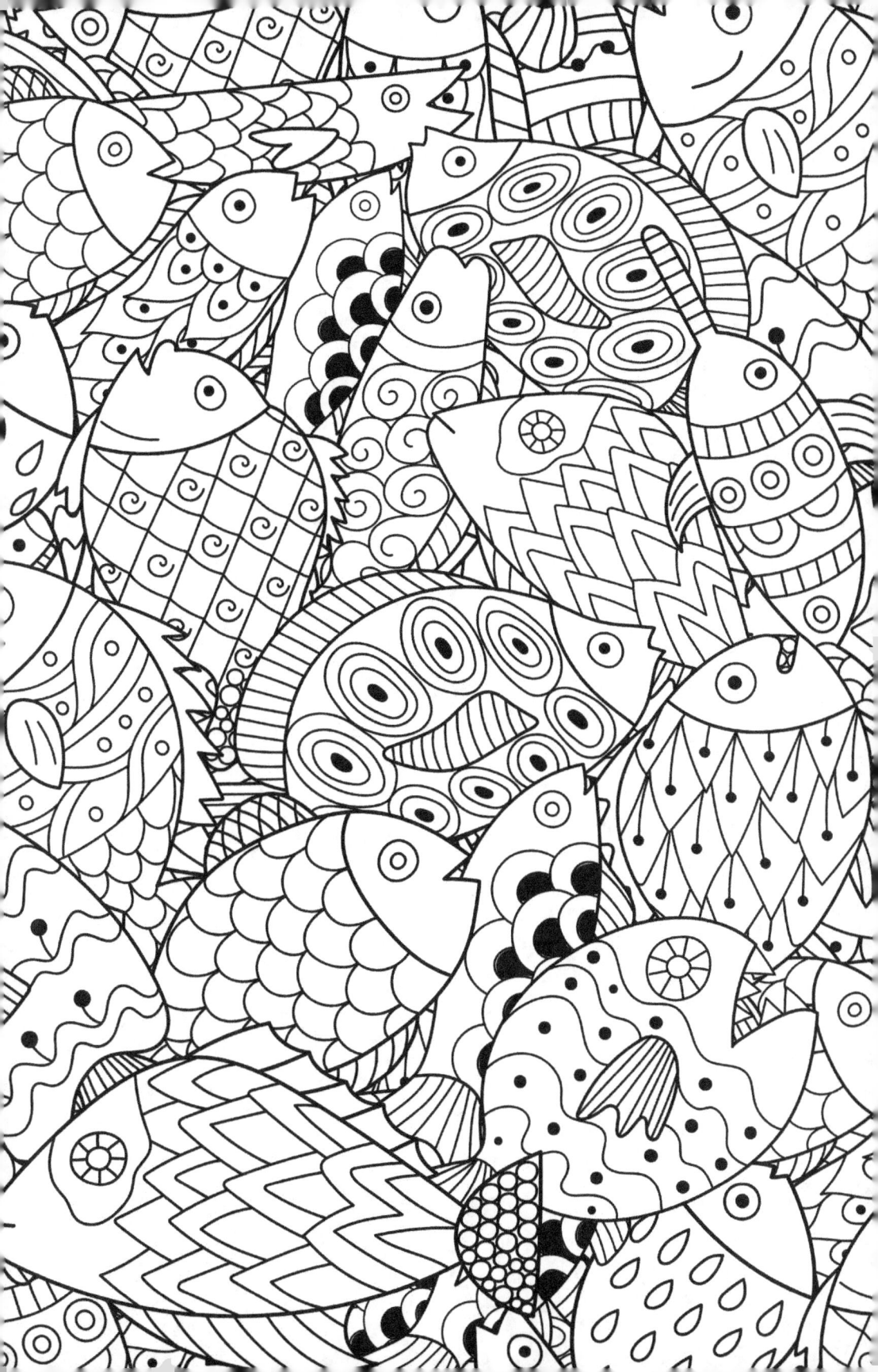

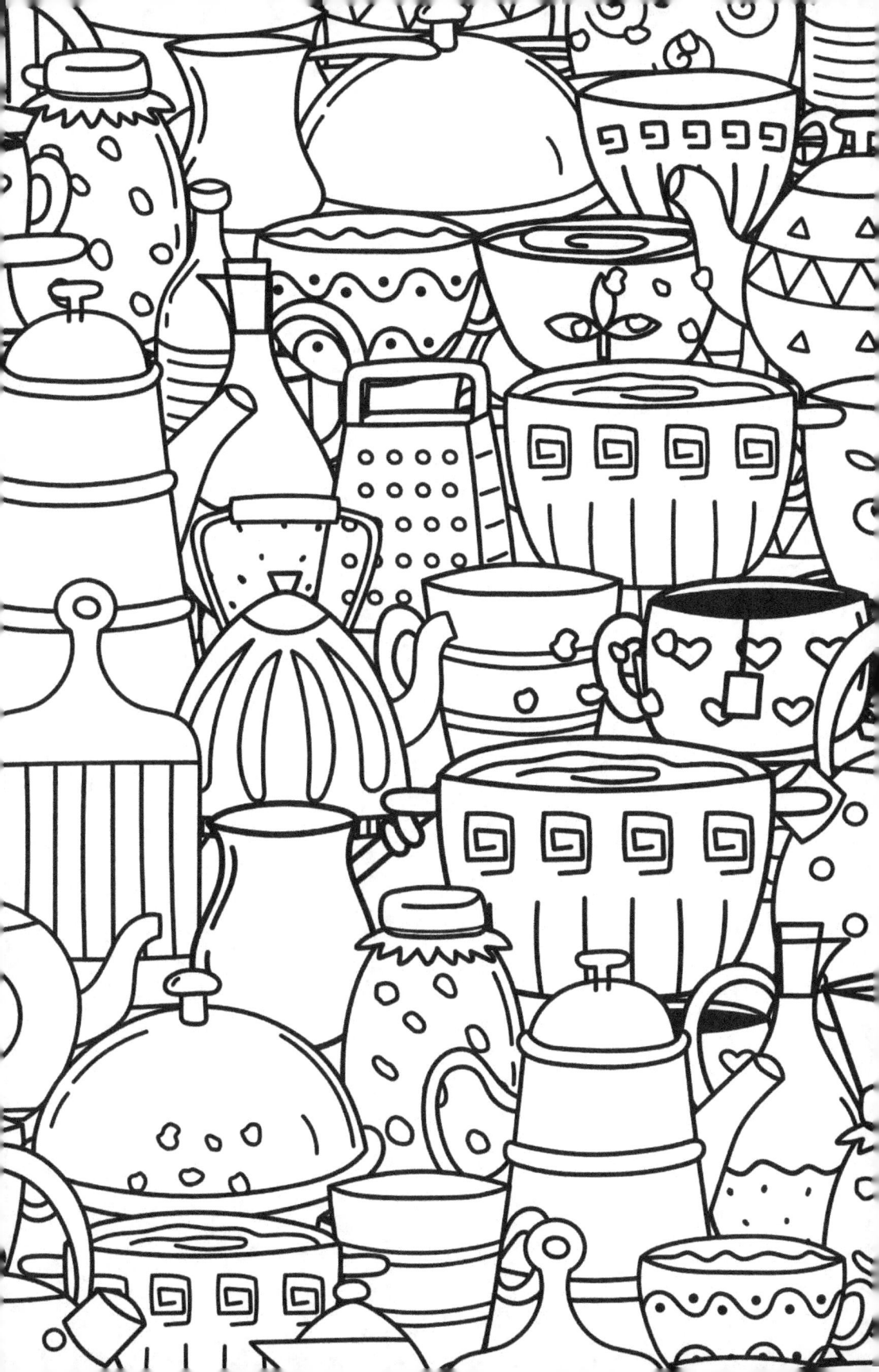

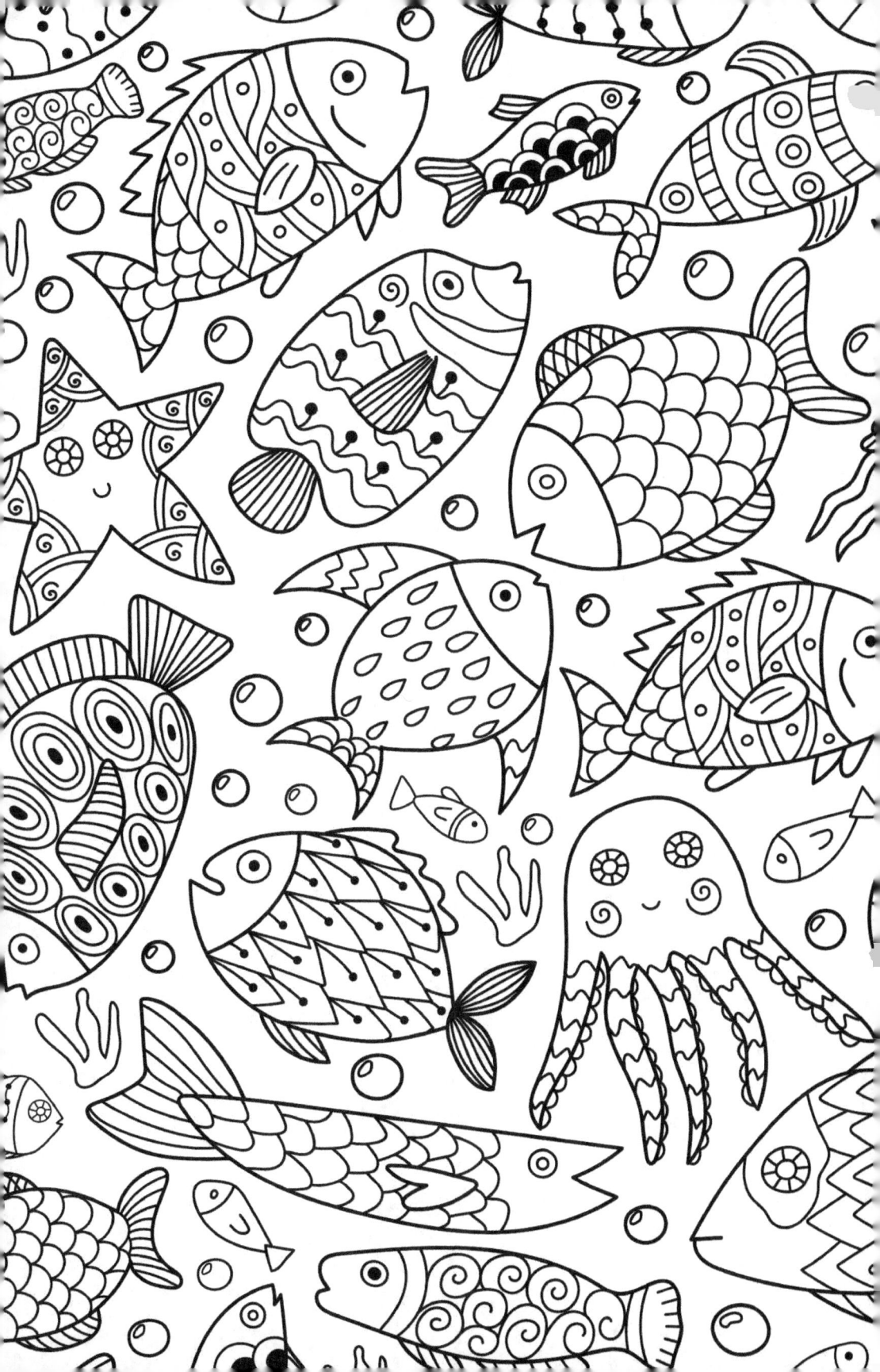

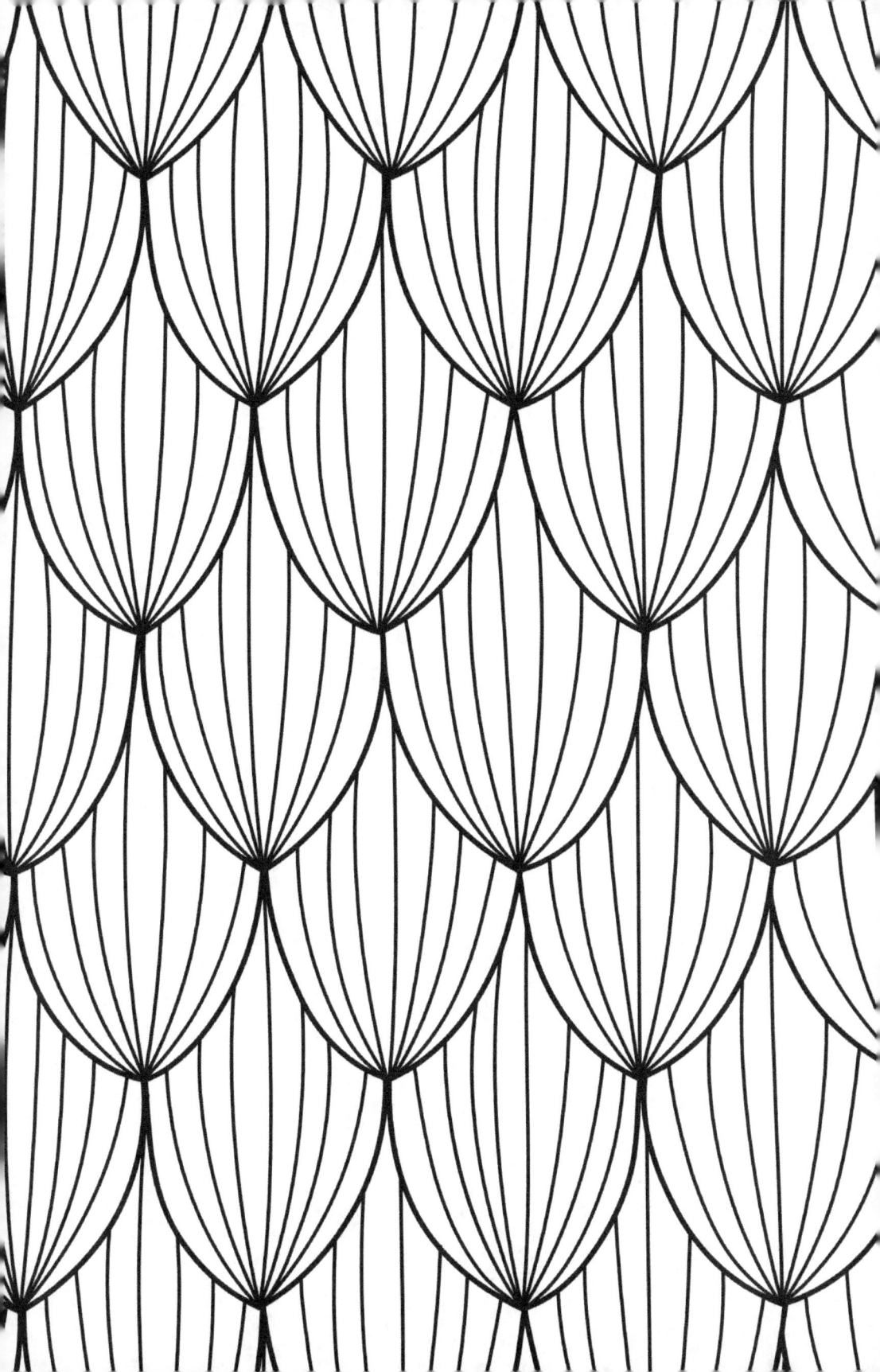

www.ingramcontent.com/pod-product-compliance
Lightning Source LLC
Chambersburg PA
CBHW070426290526
45791CB00005B/1861